Strain

I0402768

Grower _____ Date _____

Acquired _____ $ _____

| Indica | Hybrid | Sativa |

☐ Flower ☐ Edible ☐ Concentrate

Sweet · Fruity · Floral · Sour · Spicy · Earthy · Herbal · Woodsy

Symptoms Relieved
_____
_____
_____
_____

Notes
_____
_____
_____
_____
_____

Effects	Strength
Peaceful	○ ○ ○ ○ ○
Sleepy	○ ○ ○ ○ ○
Pain Relief	○ ○ ○ ○ ○
Hungry	○ ○ ○ ○ ○
Uplifted	○ ○ ○ ○ ○
Creative	○ ○ ○ ○ ○

Ratings ☆ ☆ ☆ ☆ ☆

Strain

Grower _____   Date _____

Acquired _____ $ _____

| Indica | Hybrid | Sativa |

☐ Flower   ☐ Edible   ☐ Concentrate

Symptoms Relieved

_____
_____
_____
_____
_____

Notes

_____
_____
_____
_____
_____
_____
_____

Aroma wheel: Sweet, Floral, Spicy, Herbal, Woodsy, Earthy, Sour, Fruity

Effects	Strength
Peaceful	○ ○ ○ ○ ○
Sleepy	○ ○ ○ ○ ○
Pain Relief	○ ○ ○ ○ ○
Hungry	○ ○ ○ ○ ○
Uplifted	○ ○ ○ ○ ○
Creative	○ ○ ○ ○ ○

Ratings ☆ ☆ ☆ ☆ ☆

Strain

Grower _____   Date _____

Acquired _____ $ _____

| Indica | Hybrid | Sativa |

☐ Flower   ☐ Edible   ☐ Concentrate

Symptoms Relieved

_____
_____
_____
_____
_____

Sweet · Floral · Spicy · Herbal · Woodsy · Earthy · Sour · Fruity

Notes

_____
_____
_____
_____
_____
_____

Effects	Strength				
Peaceful	○	○	○	○	○
Sleepy	○	○	○	○	○
Pain Relief	○	○	○	○	○
Hungry	○	○	○	○	○
Uplifted	○	○	○	○	○
Creative	○	○	○	○	○

Ratings ☆ ☆ ☆ ☆ ☆

Strain

Grower _____ Date _____
Acquired _____ $ _____

| Indica | Hybrid | Sativa |

☐ Flower ☐ Edible ☐ Concentrate

Sweet · Fruity · Floral · Spicy · Herbal · Woodsy · Earthy · Sour

Symptoms Relieved
_____
_____
_____
_____
_____

Notes
_____
_____
_____
_____
_____
_____

Effects	Strength				
Peaceful	○	○	○	○	○
Sleepy	○	○	○	○	○
Pain Relief	○	○	○	○	○
Hungry	○	○	○	○	○
Uplifted	○	○	○	○	○
Creative	○	○	○	○	○

Ratings ☆ ☆ ☆ ☆ ☆

Strain

Grower _____   Date _____

Acquired _____ $ _____

| Indica | Hybrid | Sativa |

☐ Flower   ☐ Edible   ☐ Concentrate

Symptoms Relieved

_____
_____
_____
_____
_____

Sweet · Fruity · Floral · Sour · Spicy · Earthy · Woodsy · Herbal

Notes

_____
_____
_____
_____
_____
_____

Effects	Strength				
Peaceful	○	○	○	○	○
Sleepy	○	○	○	○	○
Pain Relief	○	○	○	○	○
Hungry	○	○	○	○	○
Uplifted	○	○	○	○	○
Creative	○	○	○	○	○

Ratings ☆ ☆ ☆ ☆ ☆

Strain

Grower _____ Date _____

Acquired _____ $ _____

| Indica | Hybrid | Sativa |

☐ Flower ☐ Edible ☐ Concentrate

Symptoms Relieved

_____
_____
_____
_____

Sweet · Fruity · Floral · Sour · Spicy · Earthy · Woodsy · Herbal

Notes

_____
_____
_____
_____
_____
_____

Effects	Strength				
Peaceful	○	○	○	○	○
Sleepy	○	○	○	○	○
Pain Relief	○	○	○	○	○
Hungry	○	○	○	○	○
Uplifted	○	○	○	○	○
Creative	○	○	○	○	○

Ratings ☆ ☆ ☆ ☆ ☆

Strain

Grower _____   Date _____

Acquired _____ $ _____

| Indica | Hybrid | Sativa |

☐ Flower   ☐ Edible   ☐ Concentrate

Symptoms Relieved
_____
_____
_____
_____
_____

Notes
_____
_____
_____
_____
_____
_____

Flavor wheel: Sweet, Floral, Spicy, Herbal, Woodsy, Earthy, Sour, Fruity

Effects	Strength				
Peaceful	○	○	○	○	○
Sleepy	○	○	○	○	○
Pain Relief	○	○	○	○	○
Hungry	○	○	○	○	○
Uplifted	○	○	○	○	○
Creative	○	○	○	○	○

Ratings ☆ ☆ ☆ ☆ ☆

Strain

Grower _____ Date _____
Acquired _____ $ _____

Indica　　　　　　　Hybrid　　　　　　　Sativa

☐ Flower　　☐ Edible　　☐ Concentrate

Symptoms Relieved

_____
_____
_____
_____
_____

Sweet
Fruity　　Floral
Sour　　　　　Spicy
Earthy　　Herbal
Woodsy

Notes

_____
_____
_____
_____
_____
_____

Effects	Strength				
Peaceful	○	○	○	○	○
Sleepy	○	○	○	○	○
Pain Relief	○	○	○	○	○
Hungry	○	○	○	○	○
Uplifted	○	○	○	○	○
Creative	○	○	○	○	○

Ratings ☆ ☆ ☆ ☆ ☆

Strain

Grower _____ Date _____

Acquired _____ $ _____

| Indica | Hybrid | Sativa |

☐ Flower   ☐ Edible   ☐ Concentrate

Symptoms Relieved

_____
_____
_____
_____
_____

Sweet / Floral / Spicy / Herbal / Woodsy / Earthy / Sour / Fruity

Notes

_____
_____
_____
_____
_____

Effects	Strength				
Peaceful	○	○	○	○	○
Sleepy	○	○	○	○	○
Pain Relief	○	○	○	○	○
Hungry	○	○	○	○	○
Uplifted	○	○	○	○	○
Creative	○	○	○	○	○

Ratings ☆ ☆ ☆ ☆ ☆

Strain

Grower _____ Date _____

Acquired _____ $ _____

| Indica | Hybrid | Sativa |

☐ Flower ☐ Edible ☐ Concentrate

Symptoms Relieved

_____
_____
_____
_____
_____

Notes

_____
_____
_____
_____
_____
_____

Aroma wheel: Sweet, Floral, Spicy, Herbal, Woodsy, Earthy, Sour, Fruity

Effects	Strength				
Peaceful	○	○	○	○	○
Sleepy	○	○	○	○	○
Pain Relief	○	○	○	○	○
Hungry	○	○	○	○	○
Uplifted	○	○	○	○	○
Creative	○	○	○	○	○

Ratings ☆ ☆ ☆ ☆ ☆

Strain

Grower _____ Date _____

Acquired _____ $ _____

| Indica | Hybrid | Sativa |

☐ Flower   ☐ Edible   ☐ Concentrate

Symptoms Relieved

_____
_____
_____
_____

Sweet / Floral / Spicy / Herbal / Woodsy / Earthy / Sour / Fruity

Notes

_____
_____
_____
_____
_____

Effects	Strength
Peaceful	○ ○ ○ ○ ○
Sleepy	○ ○ ○ ○ ○
Pain Relief	○ ○ ○ ○ ○
Hungry	○ ○ ○ ○ ○
Uplifted	○ ○ ○ ○ ○
Creative	○ ○ ○ ○ ○

Ratings ☆ ☆ ☆ ☆ ☆

Strain

Grower _____ Date _____

Acquired _____ $ _____

| Indica | Hybrid | Sativa |

☐ Flower ☐ Edible ☐ Concentrate

Symptoms Relieved
_____
_____
_____
_____

Sweet Floral Spicy Herbal Woodsy Earthy Sour Fruity

Notes
_____
_____
_____
_____
_____
_____

Effects	Strength
Peaceful	○ ○ ○ ○ ○
Sleepy	○ ○ ○ ○ ○
Pain Relief	○ ○ ○ ○ ○
Hungry	○ ○ ○ ○ ○
Uplifted	○ ○ ○ ○ ○
Creative	○ ○ ○ ○ ○

Ratings ☆ ☆ ☆ ☆ ☆

Strain

Grower _____ Date _____

Acquired _____ $ _____

| Indica | Hybrid | Sativa |

☐ Flower ☐ Edible ☐ Concentrate

Symptoms Relieved

_____
_____
_____
_____
_____

Sweet · Floral · Spicy · Herbal · Woodsy · Earthy · Sour · Fruity

Notes

_____
_____
_____
_____
_____
_____

Effects	Strength				
Peaceful	○	○	○	○	○
Sleepy	○	○	○	○	○
Pain Relief	○	○	○	○	○
Hungry	○	○	○	○	○
Uplifted	○	○	○	○	○
Creative	○	○	○	○	○

Ratings ☆ ☆ ☆ ☆ ☆

Strain

Grower _____ Date _____

Acquired _____ $ _____

| Indica | Hybrid | Sativa |

☐ Flower   ☐ Edible   ☐ Concentrate

Symptoms Relieved

_____
_____
_____
_____
_____

Sweet / Fruity / Floral / Sour / Spicy / Earthy / Woodsy / Herbal

Notes

_____
_____
_____
_____
_____
_____
_____

Effects	Strength				
Peaceful	○	○	○	○	○
Sleepy	○	○	○	○	○
Pain Relief	○	○	○	○	○
Hungry	○	○	○	○	○
Uplifted	○	○	○	○	○
Creative	○	○	○	○	○

Ratings ☆ ☆ ☆ ☆ ☆

Strain

Grower _____   Date _____

Acquired _____ $ _____

| Indica | Hybrid | Sativa |

☐ Flower ☐ Edible ☐ Concentrate

Symptoms Relieved

_____
_____
_____
_____
_____

Sweet Floral Spicy Herbal Woodsy Earthy Sour Fruity

Notes

_____
_____
_____
_____
_____
_____
_____

Effects	Strength				
Peaceful	○	○	○	○	○
Sleepy	○	○	○	○	○
Pain Relief	○	○	○	○	○
Hungry	○	○	○	○	○
Uplifted	○	○	○	○	○
Creative	○	○	○	○	○

Ratings ☆ ☆ ☆ ☆ ☆

Strain

Grower _____ Date _____

Acquired _____ $ _____

| Indica | Hybrid | Sativa |

☐ Flower ☐ Edible ☐ Concentrate

Symptoms Relieved

_____
_____
_____
_____
_____

Sweet / Fruity / Floral / Sour / Spicy / Earthy / Woodsy / Herbal

Notes

_____
_____
_____
_____
_____

Effects	Strength				
Peaceful	○	○	○	○	○
Sleepy	○	○	○	○	○
Pain Relief	○	○	○	○	○
Hungry	○	○	○	○	○
Uplifted	○	○	○	○	○
Creative	○	○	○	○	○

Ratings ☆ ☆ ☆ ☆ ☆

Strain

Grower _____ Date _____

Acquired _____ $ _____

| Indica | Hybrid | Sativa |

☐ Flower ☐ Edible ☐ Concentrate

Symptoms Relieved

_____
_____
_____
_____
_____

Sweet · Floral · Spicy · Herbal · Woodsy · Earthy · Sour · Fruity

Notes

_____
_____
_____
_____
_____

Effects	Strength				
Peaceful	○	○	○	○	○
Sleepy	○	○	○	○	○
Pain Relief	○	○	○	○	○
Hungry	○	○	○	○	○
Uplifted	○	○	○	○	○
Creative	○	○	○	○	○

Ratings ☆ ☆ ☆ ☆ ☆

Strain

Grower _____ Date _____

Acquired _____ $ _____

| Indica | Hybrid | Sativa |

☐ Flower ☐ Edible ☐ Concentrate

Sweet / Fruity / Floral / Sour / Spicy / Earthy / Woodsy / Herbal

Symptoms Relieved

_____
_____
_____
_____
_____

Notes

_____
_____
_____
_____
_____
_____

Effects	Strength
Peaceful	○ ○ ○ ○ ○
Sleepy	○ ○ ○ ○ ○
Pain Relief	○ ○ ○ ○ ○
Hungry	○ ○ ○ ○ ○
Uplifted	○ ○ ○ ○ ○
Creative	○ ○ ○ ○ ○

Ratings ☆ ☆ ☆ ☆ ☆

Strain

Grower _____ Date _____

Acquired _____ $ _____

| Indica | Hybrid | Sativa |

☐ Flower   ☐ Edible   ☐ Concentrate

Sweet
Fruity   Floral
Sour   Spicy
Earthy   Herbal
Woodsy

Symptoms Relieved

_____
_____
_____
_____
_____

Notes

_____
_____
_____
_____
_____
_____

Effects	Strength				
Peaceful	○	○	○	○	○
Sleepy	○	○	○	○	○
Pain Relief	○	○	○	○	○
Hungry	○	○	○	○	○
Uplifted	○	○	○	○	○
Creative	○	○	○	○	○

Ratings ☆ ☆ ☆ ☆ ☆

Strain

Grower _____   Date _____

Acquired _____ $ _____

| Indica | Hybrid | Sativa |

☐ Flower   ☐ Edible   ☐ Concentrate

Symptoms Relieved

_____
_____
_____
_____

Sweet
Fruity   Floral
Sour   Spicy
Earthy   Herbal
Woodsy

Notes

_____
_____
_____
_____
_____
_____

Effects	Strength				
Peaceful	○	○	○	○	○
Sleepy	○	○	○	○	○
Pain Relief	○	○	○	○	○
Hungry	○	○	○	○	○
Uplifted	○	○	○	○	○
Creative	○	○	○	○	○

Ratings ☆ ☆ ☆ ☆ ☆

Strain

Grower _____ Date _____

Acquired _____ $ _____

| Indica | Hybrid | Sativa |

☐ Flower ☐ Edible ☐ Concentrate

Symptoms Relieved

_____
_____
_____
_____
_____

Sweet · Floral · Spicy · Herbal · Woodsy · Earthy · Sour · Fruity

Notes

_____
_____
_____
_____
_____
_____
_____

Effects	Strength				
Peaceful	○	○	○	○	○
Sleepy	○	○	○	○	○
Pain Relief	○	○	○	○	○
Hungry	○	○	○	○	○
Uplifted	○	○	○	○	○
Creative	○	○	○	○	○

Ratings ☆ ☆ ☆ ☆ ☆

Strain

Grower _____ Date _____

Acquired _____ $ _____

| Indica | Hybrid | Sativa |

☐ Flower ☐ Edible ☐ Concentrate

Symptoms Relieved

_____
_____
_____
_____
_____

Sweet / Fruity / Floral / Sour / Spicy / Earthy / Woodsy / Herbal

Notes

_____
_____
_____
_____
_____
_____

Effects	Strength				
Peaceful	○	○	○	○	○
Sleepy	○	○	○	○	○
Pain Relief	○	○	○	○	○
Hungry	○	○	○	○	○
Uplifted	○	○	○	○	○
Creative	○	○	○	○	○

Ratings ☆ ☆ ☆ ☆ ☆

Strain

Grower _____ Date _____

Acquired _____ $ _____

| Indica | Hybrid | Sativa |

☐ Flower   ☐ Edible   ☐ Concentrate

Symptoms Relieved
_____
_____
_____
_____
_____

Sweet · Fruity · Floral · Sour · Spicy · Earthy · Woodsy · Herbal

Notes
_____
_____
_____
_____
_____
_____

Effects	Strength
Peaceful	○ ○ ○ ○ ○
Sleepy	○ ○ ○ ○ ○
Pain Relief	○ ○ ○ ○ ○
Hungry	○ ○ ○ ○ ○
Uplifted	○ ○ ○ ○ ○
Creative	○ ○ ○ ○ ○

Ratings ☆ ☆ ☆ ☆ ☆

Strain

Grower _____ Date _____

Acquired _____ $ _____

Indica   Hybrid   Sativa

☐ Flower   ☐ Edible   ☐ Concentrate

Symptoms Relieved

_____
_____
_____
_____

Sweet
Fruity   Floral
Sour   Spicy
Earthy   Herbal
Woodsy

Notes

_____
_____
_____
_____
_____
_____

Effects	Strength				
Peaceful	○	○	○	○	○
Sleepy	○	○	○	○	○
Pain Relief	○	○	○	○	○
Hungry	○	○	○	○	○
Uplifted	○	○	○	○	○
Creative	○	○	○	○	○

Ratings ☆ ☆ ☆ ☆ ☆

Strain

Grower _____ Date _____

Acquired _____ $ _____

| Indica | Hybrid | Sativa |

☐ Flower ☐ Edible ☐ Concentrate

Symptoms Relieved
_____
_____
_____
_____

Sweet
Fruity
Floral
Sour
Spicy
Earthy
Herbal
Woodsy

Notes
_____
_____
_____
_____
_____
_____

Effects	Strength
Peaceful	○ ○ ○ ○ ○
Sleepy	○ ○ ○ ○ ○
Pain Relief	○ ○ ○ ○ ○
Hungry	○ ○ ○ ○ ○
Uplifted	○ ○ ○ ○ ○
Creative	○ ○ ○ ○ ○

Ratings ☆ ☆ ☆ ☆ ☆

Strain

Grower _____   Date _____

Acquired _____ $ _____

| Indica | Hybrid | Sativa |

☐ Flower ☐ Edible ☐ Concentrate

Symptoms Relieved

_____
_____
_____
_____

Sweet · Floral · Spicy · Herbal · Woodsy · Earthy · Sour · Fruity

Notes

_____
_____
_____
_____
_____
_____

Effects	Strength				
Peaceful	○	○	○	○	○
Sleepy	○	○	○	○	○
Pain Relief	○	○	○	○	○
Hungry	○	○	○	○	○
Uplifted	○	○	○	○	○
Creative	○	○	○	○	○

Ratings ☆ ☆ ☆ ☆ ☆

Strain

Grower _____ Date _____

Acquired _____ $ _____

| Indica | Hybrid | Sativa |

☐ Flower ☐ Edible ☐ Concentrate

Symptoms Relieved

_____

_____

_____

_____

_____

Flavor wheel: Sweet, Floral, Spicy, Herbal, Woodsy, Earthy, Sour, Fruity

Notes

_____

_____

_____

_____

_____

_____

Effects	Strength				
Peaceful	○	○	○	○	○
Sleepy	○	○	○	○	○
Pain Relief	○	○	○	○	○
Hungry	○	○	○	○	○
Uplifted	○	○	○	○	○
Creative	○	○	○	○	○

Ratings ☆ ☆ ☆ ☆ ☆

Strain

Grower _____ Date _____

Acquired _____ $ _____

Indica   Hybrid   Sativa

☐ Flower   ☐ Edible   ☐ Concentrate

Symptoms Relieved
_____
_____
_____
_____
_____

Sweet
Fruity   Floral
Sour   Spicy
Earthy   Herbal
Woodsy

Notes
_____
_____
_____
_____
_____
_____
_____

Effects	Strength				
Peaceful	○	○	○	○	○
Sleepy	○	○	○	○	○
Pain Relief	○	○	○	○	○
Hungry	○	○	○	○	○
Uplifted	○	○	○	○	○
Creative	○	○	○	○	○

Ratings ☆ ☆ ☆ ☆ ☆

Strain

Grower _____ Date _____

Acquired _____ $ _____

| Indica | Hybrid | Sativa |

☐ Flower ☐ Edible ☐ Concentrate

Sweet
Fruity   Floral
Sour   Spicy
Earthy   Herbal
Woodsy

Symptoms Relieved

_____
_____
_____
_____
_____

Notes

_____
_____
_____
_____
_____
_____

Effects	Strength
Peaceful	○ ○ ○ ○ ○
Sleepy	○ ○ ○ ○ ○
Pain Relief	○ ○ ○ ○ ○
Hungry	○ ○ ○ ○ ○
Uplifted	○ ○ ○ ○ ○
Creative	○ ○ ○ ○ ○

Ratings ☆ ☆ ☆ ☆ ☆

Strain

Grower _____   Date _____

Acquired _____ $ _____

| Indica | Hybrid | Sativa |

☐ Flower ☐ Edible ☐ Concentrate

Symptoms Relieved

_____
_____
_____
_____
_____

Sweet · Fruity · Floral · Sour · Spicy · Earthy · Woodsy · Herbal

Notes

_____
_____
_____
_____
_____
_____

Effects	Strength				
Peaceful	○	○	○	○	○
Sleepy	○	○	○	○	○
Pain Relief	○	○	○	○	○
Hungry	○	○	○	○	○
Uplifted	○	○	○	○	○
Creative	○	○	○	○	○

Ratings ☆ ☆ ☆ ☆ ☆

Strain

Grower _____ Date _____

Acquired _____ $ _____

| Indica | Hybrid | Sativa |

☐ Flower ☐ Edible ☐ Concentrate

Sweet
Fruity   Floral
Sour   Spicy
Earthy   Herbal
Woodsy

Symptoms Relieved
_____
_____
_____
_____
_____

Notes
_____
_____
_____
_____
_____

Effects	Strength				
Peaceful	○	○	○	○	○
Sleepy	○	○	○	○	○
Pain Relief	○	○	○	○	○
Hungry	○	○	○	○	○
Uplifted	○	○	○	○	○
Creative	○	○	○	○	○

Ratings ☆ ☆ ☆ ☆ ☆

Strain

Grower _____ Date _____

Acquired _____ $ _____

| Indica | Hybrid | Sativa |

☐ Flower   ☐ Edible   ☐ Concentrate

Symptoms Relieved

_____
_____
_____
_____

Sweet / Floral / Spicy / Herbal / Woodsy / Earthy / Sour / Fruity

Notes

_____
_____
_____
_____
_____
_____

Effects	Strength
Peaceful	○ ○ ○ ○ ○
Sleepy	○ ○ ○ ○ ○
Pain Relief	○ ○ ○ ○ ○
Hungry	○ ○ ○ ○ ○
Uplifted	○ ○ ○ ○ ○
Creative	○ ○ ○ ○ ○

Ratings ☆ ☆ ☆ ☆ ☆

Strain

Grower _____ Date _____

Acquired _____ $ _____

| Indica | Hybrid | Sativa |

☐ Flower ☐ Edible ☐ Concentrate

Sweet
Fruity Floral
Sour Spicy
Earthy Herbal
Woodsy

Symptoms Relieved

_____
_____
_____
_____
_____

Notes

_____
_____
_____
_____
_____
_____

Effects	Strength
Peaceful	○ ○ ○ ○ ○
Sleepy	○ ○ ○ ○ ○
Pain Relief	○ ○ ○ ○ ○
Hungry	○ ○ ○ ○ ○
Uplifted	○ ○ ○ ○ ○
Creative	○ ○ ○ ○ ○

Ratings ☆ ☆ ☆ ☆ ☆

Strain

Grower _____ Date _____

Acquired _____ $ _____

| Indica | Hybrid | Sativa |

☐ Flower ☐ Edible ☐ Concentrate

Symptoms Relieved

_____
_____
_____
_____
_____

Sweet / Floral / Spicy / Herbal / Woodsy / Earthy / Sour / Fruity

Notes

_____
_____
_____
_____
_____
_____

Effects	Strength				
Peaceful	○	○	○	○	○
Sleepy	○	○	○	○	○
Pain Relief	○	○	○	○	○
Hungry	○	○	○	○	○
Uplifted	○	○	○	○	○
Creative	○	○	○	○	○

Ratings ☆ ☆ ☆ ☆ ☆

Strain

Grower _____   Date _____

Acquired _____ $ _____

| Indica | Hybrid | Sativa |

☐ Flower   ☐ Edible   ☐ Concentrate

Symptoms Relieved

_____
_____
_____
_____
_____

Sweet · Floral · Spicy · Herbal · Woodsy · Earthy · Sour · Fruity

Notes

_____
_____
_____
_____
_____
_____

Effects	Strength				
Peaceful	○	○	○	○	○
Sleepy	○	○	○	○	○
Pain Relief	○	○	○	○	○
Hungry	○	○	○	○	○
Uplifted	○	○	○	○	○
Creative	○	○	○	○	○

Ratings ☆ ☆ ☆ ☆ ☆

Strain

Grower _____ Date _____

Acquired _____ $ _____

| Indica | Hybrid | Sativa |

☐ Flower ☐ Edible ☐ Concentrate

```
         Sweet
 Fruity        Floral

Sour             Spicy

 Earthy        Herbal
        Woodsy
```

Symptoms Relieved

_____
_____
_____
_____
_____

Notes

_____
_____
_____
_____
_____
_____

Effects	Strength
Peaceful	○ ○ ○ ○ ○
Sleepy	○ ○ ○ ○ ○
Pain Relief	○ ○ ○ ○ ○
Hungry	○ ○ ○ ○ ○
Uplifted	○ ○ ○ ○ ○
Creative	○ ○ ○ ○ ○

Ratings ☆ ☆ ☆ ☆ ☆

Strain

Grower _____ Date _____

Acquired _____ $ _____

| Indica | Hybrid | Sativa |

☐ Flower ☐ Edible ☐ Concentrate

Symptoms Relieved
_____
_____
_____
_____
_____

Sweet · Floral · Spicy · Herbal · Woodsy · Earthy · Sour · Fruity

Notes
_____
_____
_____
_____
_____

Effects	Strength				
Peaceful	○	○	○	○	○
Sleepy	○	○	○	○	○
Pain Relief	○	○	○	○	○
Hungry	○	○	○	○	○
Uplifted	○	○	○	○	○
Creative	○	○	○	○	○

Ratings ☆ ☆ ☆ ☆ ☆

Strain

Grower _____   Date _____

Acquired _____ $ _____

| Indica | Hybrid | Sativa |

☐ Flower   ☐ Edible   ☐ Concentrate

Symptoms Relieved

_____
_____
_____
_____

Sweet / Fruity / Floral / Sour / Spicy / Earthy / Woodsy / Herbal

Notes

_____
_____
_____
_____
_____
_____

Effects	Strength
Peaceful	○ ○ ○ ○ ○
Sleepy	○ ○ ○ ○ ○
Pain Relief	○ ○ ○ ○ ○
Hungry	○ ○ ○ ○ ○
Uplifted	○ ○ ○ ○ ○
Creative	○ ○ ○ ○ ○

Ratings ☆ ☆ ☆ ☆ ☆

Strain

Grower _____ Date _____

Acquired _____ $ _____

| Indica | Hybrid | Sativa |

☐ Flower ☐ Edible ☐ Concentrate

Sweet
Fruity   Floral
Sour   Spicy
Earthy   Herbal
Woodsy

Symptoms Relieved

_____
_____
_____
_____
_____

Notes

_____
_____
_____
_____
_____
_____

Effects	Strength				
Peaceful	○	○	○	○	○
Sleepy	○	○	○	○	○
Pain Relief	○	○	○	○	○
Hungry	○	○	○	○	○
Uplifted	○	○	○	○	○
Creative	○	○	○	○	○

Ratings ☆ ☆ ☆ ☆ ☆

Strain

Grower _____ Date _____

Acquired _____ $ _____

| Indica | Hybrid | Sativa |

☐ Flower   ☐ Edible   ☐ Concentrate

Sweet · Fruity · Floral · Sour · Spicy · Earthy · Woodsy · Herbal

Symptoms Relieved

_____
_____
_____
_____
_____

Notes

_____
_____
_____
_____
_____
_____

Effects	Strength				
Peaceful	○	○	○	○	○
Sleepy	○	○	○	○	○
Pain Relief	○	○	○	○	○
Hungry	○	○	○	○	○
Uplifted	○	○	○	○	○
Creative	○	○	○	○	○

Ratings ☆ ☆ ☆ ☆ ☆

Strain

Grower _____ Date _____

Acquired _____ $ _____

| Indica | Hybrid | Sativa |

☐ Flower ☐ Edible ☐ Concentrate

Symptoms Relieved
_____
_____
_____
_____
_____

Sweet · Floral · Spicy · Herbal · Woodsy · Earthy · Sour · Fruity

Notes
_____
_____
_____
_____
_____
_____

Effects	Strength				
Peaceful	○	○	○	○	○
Sleepy	○	○	○	○	○
Pain Relief	○	○	○	○	○
Hungry	○	○	○	○	○
Uplifted	○	○	○	○	○
Creative	○	○	○	○	○

Ratings ☆ ☆ ☆ ☆ ☆

Strain

Grower _____ Date _____

Acquired _____ $ _____

| Indica | Hybrid | Sativa |

☐ Flower ☐ Edible ☐ Concentrate

Sweet / Fruity / Floral / Sour / Spicy / Earthy / Woodsy / Herbal

Symptoms Relieved

_____
_____
_____
_____

Notes

_____
_____
_____
_____
_____

Effects	Strength
Peaceful	○ ○ ○ ○ ○
Sleepy	○ ○ ○ ○ ○
Pain Relief	○ ○ ○ ○ ○
Hungry	○ ○ ○ ○ ○
Uplifted	○ ○ ○ ○ ○
Creative	○ ○ ○ ○ ○

Ratings ☆ ☆ ☆ ☆ ☆

Strain

Grower _____ Date _____

Acquired _____ $ _____

| Indica | Hybrid | Sativa |

☐ Flower ☐ Edible ☐ Concentrate

Sweet
Fruity Floral
Sour Spicy
Earthy Herbal
Woodsy

Symptoms Relieved

_____
_____
_____
_____
_____

Notes

_____
_____
_____
_____
_____
_____

Effects	Strength				
Peaceful	○	○	○	○	○
Sleepy	○	○	○	○	○
Pain Relief	○	○	○	○	○
Hungry	○	○	○	○	○
Uplifted	○	○	○	○	○
Creative	○	○	○	○	○

Ratings ☆ ☆ ☆ ☆ ☆

Strain

Grower _____ Date _____

Acquired _____ $ _____

| Indica | Hybrid | Sativa |

☐ Flower ☐ Edible ☐ Concentrate

Symptoms Relieved

_____
_____
_____
_____
_____

Sweet · Floral · Spicy · Herbal · Woodsy · Earthy · Sour · Fruity

Notes

_____
_____
_____
_____
_____
_____

Effects	Strength				
Peaceful	○	○	○	○	○
Sleepy	○	○	○	○	○
Pain Relief	○	○	○	○	○
Hungry	○	○	○	○	○
Uplifted	○	○	○	○	○
Creative	○	○	○	○	○

Ratings ☆ ☆ ☆ ☆ ☆

Strain

Grower _____ Date _____

Acquired _____ $ _____

| Indica | Hybrid | Sativa |

☐ Flower   ☐ Edible   ☐ Concentrate

Symptoms Relieved

_____
_____
_____
_____
_____

Sweet · Floral · Spicy · Herbal · Woodsy · Earthy · Sour · Fruity

Notes

_____
_____
_____
_____
_____
_____

Effects	Strength				
Peaceful	○	○	○	○	○
Sleepy	○	○	○	○	○
Pain Relief	○	○	○	○	○
Hungry	○	○	○	○	○
Uplifted	○	○	○	○	○
Creative	○	○	○	○	○

Ratings ☆ ☆ ☆ ☆ ☆

Strain

Grower _____ Date _____

Acquired _____ $ _____

| Indica | Hybrid | Sativa |

☐ Flower ☐ Edible ☐ Concentrate

Symptoms Relieved

_____
_____
_____
_____
_____

Notes

_____
_____
_____
_____
_____
_____

Sweet / Floral / Spicy / Herbal / Woodsy / Earthy / Sour / Fruity

Effects	Strength
Peaceful	○ ○ ○ ○ ○
Sleepy	○ ○ ○ ○ ○
Pain Relief	○ ○ ○ ○ ○
Hungry	○ ○ ○ ○ ○
Uplifted	○ ○ ○ ○ ○
Creative	○ ○ ○ ○ ○

Ratings ☆ ☆ ☆ ☆ ☆

Strain

Grower _____ Date _____

Acquired _____ $ _____

| Indica | Hybrid | Sativa |

☐ Flower ☐ Edible ☐ Concentrate

Symptoms Relieved
_____
_____
_____
_____
_____

Sweet / Fruity / Floral / Sour / Spicy / Earthy / Woodsy / Herbal

Notes
_____
_____
_____
_____
_____
_____
_____

Effects	Strength				
Peaceful	○	○	○	○	○
Sleepy	○	○	○	○	○
Pain Relief	○	○	○	○	○
Hungry	○	○	○	○	○
Uplifted	○	○	○	○	○
Creative	○	○	○	○	○

Ratings ☆ ☆ ☆ ☆ ☆

Strain

Grower _____ Date _____

Acquired _____ $ _____

Indica   Hybrid   Sativa

☐ Flower   ☐ Edible   ☐ Concentrate

Sweet · Fruity · Floral · Sour · Spicy · Earthy · Woodsy · Herbal

Symptoms Relieved

_____
_____
_____
_____

Notes

_____
_____
_____
_____
_____

Effects	Strength				
Peaceful	○	○	○	○	○
Sleepy	○	○	○	○	○
Pain Relief	○	○	○	○	○
Hungry	○	○	○	○	○
Uplifted	○	○	○	○	○
Creative	○	○	○	○	○

Ratings ☆ ☆ ☆ ☆ ☆

Strain

Grower _____ Date _____

Acquired _____ $ _____

| Indica | Hybrid | Sativa |

☐ Flower ☐ Edible ☐ Concentrate

Symptoms Relieved

_____
_____
_____
_____
_____

Sweet · Floral · Spicy · Herbal · Woodsy · Earthy · Sour · Fruity

Notes

_____
_____
_____
_____
_____
_____

Effects	Strength				
Peaceful	○	○	○	○	○
Sleepy	○	○	○	○	○
Pain Relief	○	○	○	○	○
Hungry	○	○	○	○	○
Uplifted	○	○	○	○	○
Creative	○	○	○	○	○

Ratings ☆ ☆ ☆ ☆ ☆

Strain

Grower _____ Date _____

Acquired _____ $ _____

| Indica | Hybrid | Sativa |

☐ Flower ☐ Edible ☐ Concentrate

Symptoms Relieved

_____
_____
_____
_____

Sweet / Floral / Spicy / Herbal / Woodsy / Earthy / Sour / Fruity

Notes

_____
_____
_____
_____
_____

Effects	Strength
Peaceful	○ ○ ○ ○ ○
Sleepy	○ ○ ○ ○ ○
Pain Relief	○ ○ ○ ○ ○
Hungry	○ ○ ○ ○ ○
Uplifted	○ ○ ○ ○ ○
Creative	○ ○ ○ ○ ○

Ratings ☆ ☆ ☆ ☆ ☆

Strain

Grower _____ Date _____

Acquired _____ $ _____

| Indica | Hybrid | Sativa |

☐ Flower   ☐ Edible   ☐ Concentrate

Symptoms Relieved

_____
_____
_____
_____

Sweet
Fruity   Floral
Sour   Spicy
Earthy   Herbal
Woodsy

Notes

_____
_____
_____
_____
_____

Effects	Strength				
Peaceful	○	○	○	○	○
Sleepy	○	○	○	○	○
Pain Relief	○	○	○	○	○
Hungry	○	○	○	○	○
Uplifted	○	○	○	○	○
Creative	○	○	○	○	○

Ratings ☆ ☆ ☆ ☆ ☆

Strain

Grower _____ Date _____

Acquired _____ $ _____

| Indica | Hybrid | Sativa |

☐ Flower   ☐ Edible   ☐ Concentrate

Sweet · Fruity · Floral · Sour · Spicy · Earthy · Herbal · Woodsy

Symptoms Relieved

_____
_____
_____
_____

Notes

_____
_____
_____
_____
_____

Effects	Strength
Peaceful	○ ○ ○ ○ ○
Sleepy	○ ○ ○ ○ ○
Pain Relief	○ ○ ○ ○ ○
Hungry	○ ○ ○ ○ ○
Uplifted	○ ○ ○ ○ ○
Creative	○ ○ ○ ○ ○

Ratings ☆ ☆ ☆ ☆ ☆

Strain

Grower _____ Date _____

Acquired _____ $ _____

| Indica | Hybrid | Sativa |

☐ Flower   ☐ Edible   ☐ Concentrate

Symptoms Relieved

_____
_____
_____
_____
_____

Sweet · Floral · Spicy · Herbal · Woodsy · Earthy · Sour · Fruity

Notes

_____
_____
_____
_____
_____
_____

Effects	Strength				
Peaceful	○	○	○	○	○
Sleepy	○	○	○	○	○
Pain Relief	○	○	○	○	○
Hungry	○	○	○	○	○
Uplifted	○	○	○	○	○
Creative	○	○	○	○	○

Ratings ☆ ☆ ☆ ☆ ☆

Strain

Grower _____   Date _____

Acquired _____ $ _____

| Indica | Hybrid | Sativa |

☐ Flower ☐ Edible ☐ Concentrate

Sweet Fruity Floral Sour Spicy Earthy Woodsy Herbal

Symptoms Relieved

_____
_____
_____
_____
_____

Notes

_____
_____
_____
_____
_____
_____

Effects	Strength
Peaceful	○ ○ ○ ○ ○
Sleepy	○ ○ ○ ○ ○
Pain Relief	○ ○ ○ ○ ○
Hungry	○ ○ ○ ○ ○
Uplifted	○ ○ ○ ○ ○
Creative	○ ○ ○ ○ ○

Ratings ☆ ☆ ☆ ☆ ☆

Strain

Grower _____ Date _____

Acquired _____ $ _____

Indica   Hybrid   Sativa

☐ Flower   ☐ Edible   ☐ Concentrate

Sweet, Fruity, Floral, Sour, Spicy, Earthy, Woodsy, Herbal

Symptoms Relieved

_____
_____
_____
_____
_____

Notes

_____
_____
_____
_____
_____
_____

Effects	Strength				
Peaceful	○	○	○	○	○
Sleepy	○	○	○	○	○
Pain Relief	○	○	○	○	○
Hungry	○	○	○	○	○
Uplifted	○	○	○	○	○
Creative	○	○	○	○	○

Ratings ☆ ☆ ☆ ☆ ☆

Strain

Grower _____ Date _____

Acquired _____ $ _____

Indica   Hybrid   Sativa

☐ Flower   ☐ Edible   ☐ Concentrate

Symptoms Relieved

_____
_____
_____
_____
_____

Notes

_____
_____
_____
_____
_____
_____

Sweet · Fruity · Floral · Sour · Spicy · Earthy · Woodsy · Herbal

Effects	Strength				
Peaceful	○	○	○	○	○
Sleepy	○	○	○	○	○
Pain Relief	○	○	○	○	○
Hungry	○	○	○	○	○
Uplifted	○	○	○	○	○
Creative	○	○	○	○	○

Ratings ☆ ☆ ☆ ☆ ☆

Strain

Grower _____ Date _____

Acquired _____ $ _____

| Indica | Hybrid | Sativa |

☐ Flower ☐ Edible ☐ Concentrate

Symptoms Relieved

_____
_____
_____
_____
_____

Sweet / Floral / Spicy / Herbal / Woodsy / Earthy / Sour / Fruity

Notes

_____
_____
_____
_____
_____
_____

Effects	Strength
Peaceful	○ ○ ○ ○ ○
Sleepy	○ ○ ○ ○ ○
Pain Relief	○ ○ ○ ○ ○
Hungry	○ ○ ○ ○ ○
Uplifted	○ ○ ○ ○ ○
Creative	○ ○ ○ ○ ○

Ratings ☆ ☆ ☆ ☆ ☆

Strain

Grower _____   Date _____

Acquired _____ $ _____

| Indica   Hybrid   Sativa |

☐ Flower   ☐ Edible   ☐ Concentrate

Symptoms Relieved

_____
_____
_____
_____
_____

Notes

_____
_____
_____
_____
_____
_____

Sweet · Fruity · Floral · Sour · Spicy · Earthy · Woodsy · Herbal

Effects	Strength				
Peaceful	○	○	○	○	○
Sleepy	○	○	○	○	○
Pain Relief	○	○	○	○	○
Hungry	○	○	○	○	○
Uplifted	○	○	○	○	○
Creative	○	○	○	○	○

Ratings ☆ ☆ ☆ ☆ ☆

Strain

Grower _____ Date _____

Acquired _____ $ _____

| Indica | Hybrid | Sativa |

☐ Flower ☐ Edible ☐ Concentrate

Symptoms Relieved

_____
_____
_____
_____

Sweet · Fruity · Floral · Sour · Spicy · Earthy · Herbal · Woodsy

Notes

_____
_____
_____
_____
_____

Effects	Strength				
Peaceful	○	○	○	○	○
Sleepy	○	○	○	○	○
Pain Relief	○	○	○	○	○
Hungry	○	○	○	○	○
Uplifted	○	○	○	○	○
Creative	○	○	○	○	○

Ratings ☆ ☆ ☆ ☆ ☆

Strain

Grower _____ Date _____

Acquired _____ $ _____

Indica   Hybrid   Sativa

☐ Flower   ☐ Edible   ☐ Concentrate

Symptoms Relieved

_____
_____
_____
_____

Sweet / Fruity / Floral / Sour / Spicy / Earthy / Woodsy / Herbal

Notes

_____
_____
_____
_____
_____
_____

Effects	Strength				
Peaceful	○	○	○	○	○
Sleepy	○	○	○	○	○
Pain Relief	○	○	○	○	○
Hungry	○	○	○	○	○
Uplifted	○	○	○	○	○
Creative	○	○	○	○	○

Ratings ☆ ☆ ☆ ☆ ☆

Strain

Grower _____ Date _____

Acquired _____ $ _____

| Indica | Hybrid | Sativa |

☐ Flower ☐ Edible ☐ Concentrate

Symptoms Relieved
_____
_____
_____
_____
_____

Flavor wheel: Sweet, Floral, Spicy, Herbal, Woodsy, Earthy, Sour, Fruity

Notes
_____
_____
_____
_____
_____
_____

Effects	Strength
Peaceful	○ ○ ○ ○ ○
Sleepy	○ ○ ○ ○ ○
Pain Relief	○ ○ ○ ○ ○
Hungry	○ ○ ○ ○ ○
Uplifted	○ ○ ○ ○ ○
Creative	○ ○ ○ ○ ○

Ratings ☆ ☆ ☆ ☆ ☆

Strain

Grower _____ Date _____

Acquired _____ $ _____

| Indica | Hybrid | Sativa |

☐ Flower   ☐ Edible   ☐ Concentrate

Sweet
Fruity — Floral
Sour — Spicy
Earthy — Herbal
Woodsy

Symptoms Relieved

_____
_____
_____
_____
_____

Notes

_____
_____
_____
_____
_____
_____

Effects	Strength				
Peaceful	○	○	○	○	○
Sleepy	○	○	○	○	○
Pain Relief	○	○	○	○	○
Hungry	○	○	○	○	○
Uplifted	○	○	○	○	○
Creative	○	○	○	○	○

Ratings ☆ ☆ ☆ ☆ ☆

Strain

Grower _____ Date _____

Acquired _____ $ _____

| Indica | Hybrid | Sativa |

☐ Flower ☐ Edible ☐ Concentrate

Symptoms Relieved

_____
_____
_____
_____
_____

Sweet / Floral / Spicy / Herbal / Woodsy / Earthy / Sour / Fruity

Notes

_____
_____
_____
_____
_____
_____
_____

Effects	Strength				
Peaceful	○	○	○	○	○
Sleepy	○	○	○	○	○
Pain Relief	○	○	○	○	○
Hungry	○	○	○	○	○
Uplifted	○	○	○	○	○
Creative	○	○	○	○	○

Ratings ☆ ☆ ☆ ☆ ☆

Strain

Grower _____ Date _____

Acquired _____ $ _____

| Indica | Hybrid | Sativa |

☐ Flower ☐ Edible ☐ Concentrate

Symptoms Relieved

_____
_____
_____
_____
_____

Sweet · Fruity · Floral · Sour · Spicy · Earthy · Woodsy · Herbal

Notes

_____
_____
_____
_____
_____
_____

Effects	Strength
Peaceful	○ ○ ○ ○ ○
Sleepy	○ ○ ○ ○ ○
Pain Relief	○ ○ ○ ○ ○
Hungry	○ ○ ○ ○ ○
Uplifted	○ ○ ○ ○ ○
Creative	○ ○ ○ ○ ○

Ratings ☆ ☆ ☆ ☆ ☆

Strain

Grower _____ Date _____

Acquired _____ $ _____

| Indica | Hybrid | Sativa |

☐ Flower ☐ Edible ☐ Concentrate

Symptoms Relieved
_____
_____
_____
_____

Sweet / Floral / Spicy / Herbal / Woodsy / Earthy / Sour / Fruity

Notes
_____
_____
_____
_____
_____

Effects	Strength
Peaceful	○ ○ ○ ○ ○
Sleepy	○ ○ ○ ○ ○
Pain Relief	○ ○ ○ ○ ○
Hungry	○ ○ ○ ○ ○
Uplifted	○ ○ ○ ○ ○
Creative	○ ○ ○ ○ ○

Ratings ☆ ☆ ☆ ☆ ☆

Strain

Grower _____ Date _____

Acquired _____ $ _____

| Indica | Hybrid | Sativa |

☐ Flower ☐ Edible ☐ Concentrate

Symptoms Relieved

_____
_____
_____
_____

Sweet
Fruity   Floral

Sour   Spicy

Earthy   Herbal
Woodsy

Notes

_____
_____
_____
_____
_____
_____

Effects	Strength				
Peaceful	○	○	○	○	○
Sleepy	○	○	○	○	○
Pain Relief	○	○	○	○	○
Hungry	○	○	○	○	○
Uplifted	○	○	○	○	○
Creative	○	○	○	○	○

Ratings ☆ ☆ ☆ ☆ ☆

Strain

Grower _____   Date _____

Acquired _____ $ _____

| Indica | Hybrid | Sativa |

☐ Flower   ☐ Edible   ☐ Concentrate

Symptoms Relieved

_____
_____
_____
_____
_____

Sweet / Floral / Spicy / Herbal / Woodsy / Earthy / Sour / Fruity

Notes

_____
_____
_____
_____
_____
_____
_____

Effects	Strength
Peaceful	○ ○ ○ ○ ○
Sleepy	○ ○ ○ ○ ○
Pain Relief	○ ○ ○ ○ ○
Hungry	○ ○ ○ ○ ○
Uplifted	○ ○ ○ ○ ○
Creative	○ ○ ○ ○ ○

Ratings ☆ ☆ ☆ ☆ ☆

Strain

Grower _____ Date _____

Acquired _____ $ _____

| Indica | Hybrid | Sativa |

☐ Flower ☐ Edible ☐ Concentrate

Symptoms Relieved

_____
_____
_____
_____
_____

Sweet · Floral · Spicy · Herbal · Woodsy · Earthy · Sour · Fruity

Notes

_____
_____
_____
_____
_____
_____

Effects	Strength				
Peaceful	○	○	○	○	○
Sleepy	○	○	○	○	○
Pain Relief	○	○	○	○	○
Hungry	○	○	○	○	○
Uplifted	○	○	○	○	○
Creative	○	○	○	○	○

Ratings ☆ ☆ ☆ ☆ ☆

Strain

Grower _____ Date _____

Acquired _____ $ _____

| Indica | Hybrid | Sativa |

☐ Flower ☐ Edible ☐ Concentrate

Symptoms Relieved

_____
_____
_____
_____
_____

Sweet · Floral · Spicy · Herbal · Woodsy · Earthy · Sour · Fruity

Notes

_____
_____
_____
_____
_____
_____

Effects	Strength				
Peaceful	○	○	○	○	○
Sleepy	○	○	○	○	○
Pain Relief	○	○	○	○	○
Hungry	○	○	○	○	○
Uplifted	○	○	○	○	○
Creative	○	○	○	○	○

Ratings ☆ ☆ ☆ ☆ ☆

Strain

Grower _____   Date _____

Acquired _____ $ _____

| Indica | Hybrid | Sativa |

☐ Flower   ☐ Edible   ☐ Concentrate

Symptoms Relieved

_____
_____
_____
_____

Sweet / Fruity / Floral / Sour / Spicy / Earthy / Woodsy / Herbal

Notes

_____
_____
_____
_____
_____
_____

Effects	Strength
Peaceful	○ ○ ○ ○ ○
Sleepy	○ ○ ○ ○ ○
Pain Relief	○ ○ ○ ○ ○
Hungry	○ ○ ○ ○ ○
Uplifted	○ ○ ○ ○ ○
Creative	○ ○ ○ ○ ○

Ratings ☆ ☆ ☆ ☆ ☆

Strain

Grower _____ Date _____

Acquired _____ $ _____

| Indica | Hybrid | Sativa |

☐ Flower ☐ Edible ☐ Concentrate

Symptoms Relieved
_____
_____
_____
_____

Sweet
Fruity — Floral
Sour — Spicy
Earthy — Herbal
Woodsy

Notes
_____
_____
_____
_____
_____

Effects	Strength
Peaceful	○ ○ ○ ○ ○
Sleepy	○ ○ ○ ○ ○
Pain Relief	○ ○ ○ ○ ○
Hungry	○ ○ ○ ○ ○
Uplifted	○ ○ ○ ○ ○
Creative	○ ○ ○ ○ ○

Ratings ☆ ☆ ☆ ☆ ☆

Strain

Grower _____ Date _____

Acquired _____ $ _____

| Indica | Hybrid | Sativa |

☐ Flower   ☐ Edible   ☐ Concentrate

Symptoms Relieved

_____
_____
_____
_____
_____

Sweet / Floral / Spicy / Herbal / Woodsy / Earthy / Sour / Fruity

Notes

_____
_____
_____
_____
_____
_____
_____

Effects	Strength
Peaceful	○ ○ ○ ○ ○
Sleepy	○ ○ ○ ○ ○
Pain Relief	○ ○ ○ ○ ○
Hungry	○ ○ ○ ○ ○
Uplifted	○ ○ ○ ○ ○
Creative	○ ○ ○ ○ ○

Ratings ☆ ☆ ☆ ☆ ☆

Strain

Grower _____ Date _____

Acquired _____ $ _____

| Indica | Hybrid | Sativa |

☐ Flower ☐ Edible ☐ Concentrate

Symptoms Relieved
_____
_____
_____
_____
_____

Sweet · Floral · Spicy · Herbal · Woodsy · Earthy · Sour · Fruity

Notes
_____
_____
_____
_____
_____
_____

Effects	Strength				
Peaceful	○	○	○	○	○
Sleepy	○	○	○	○	○
Pain Relief	○	○	○	○	○
Hungry	○	○	○	○	○
Uplifted	○	○	○	○	○
Creative	○	○	○	○	○

Ratings ☆ ☆ ☆ ☆ ☆

Strain

Grower _____ Date _____

Acquired _____ $ _____

| Indica | Hybrid | Sativa |

☐ Flower   ☐ Edible   ☐ Concentrate

Sweet · Fruity · Floral · Sour · Spicy · Earthy · Woodsy · Herbal

Symptoms Relieved

_____
_____
_____
_____
_____

Notes

_____
_____
_____
_____
_____
_____

Effects	Strength
Peaceful	○ ○ ○ ○ ○
Sleepy	○ ○ ○ ○ ○
Pain Relief	○ ○ ○ ○ ○
Hungry	○ ○ ○ ○ ○
Uplifted	○ ○ ○ ○ ○
Creative	○ ○ ○ ○ ○

Ratings ☆ ☆ ☆ ☆ ☆

Strain

Grower _____ Date _____

Acquired _____ $ _____

Indica   Hybrid   Sativa

☐ Flower   ☐ Edible   ☐ Concentrate

Symptoms Relieved
_____
_____
_____
_____
_____

Sweet / Floral / Spicy / Herbal / Woodsy / Earthy / Sour / Fruity

Notes
_____
_____
_____
_____
_____

Effects	Strength				
Peaceful	○	○	○	○	○
Sleepy	○	○	○	○	○
Pain Relief	○	○	○	○	○
Hungry	○	○	○	○	○
Uplifted	○	○	○	○	○
Creative	○	○	○	○	○

Ratings ☆ ☆ ☆ ☆ ☆

Strain

Grower _____ Date _____

Acquired _____ $ _____

| Indica | Hybrid | Sativa |

☐ Flower ☐ Edible ☐ Concentrate

Sweet · Fruity · Floral · Sour · Spicy · Earthy · Herbal · Woodsy

Symptoms Relieved

_____
_____
_____
_____
_____

Notes

_____
_____
_____
_____
_____
_____
_____

Effects — **Strength**

Effect					
Peaceful	○	○	○	○	○
Sleepy	○	○	○	○	○
Pain Relief	○	○	○	○	○
Hungry	○	○	○	○	○
Uplifted	○	○	○	○	○
Creative	○	○	○	○	○

Ratings ☆ ☆ ☆ ☆ ☆

Strain

Grower _____   Date _____

Acquired _____ $ _____

| Indica | Hybrid | Sativa |

☐ Flower   ☐ Edible   ☐ Concentrate

Sweet · Floral · Spicy · Herbal · Woodsy · Earthy · Sour · Fruity

Symptoms Relieved

_____
_____
_____
_____

Notes

_____
_____
_____
_____
_____

Effects	Strength
Peaceful	○ ○ ○ ○ ○
Sleepy	○ ○ ○ ○ ○
Pain Relief	○ ○ ○ ○ ○
Hungry	○ ○ ○ ○ ○
Uplifted	○ ○ ○ ○ ○
Creative	○ ○ ○ ○ ○

Ratings ☆ ☆ ☆ ☆ ☆

Strain

Grower _____ Date _____

Acquired _____ $ _____

Indica   Hybrid   Sativa

☐ Flower   ☐ Edible   ☐ Concentrate

Symptoms Relieved

_____
_____
_____
_____
_____

Notes

_____
_____
_____
_____
_____
_____

Sweet / Fruity / Floral / Sour / Spicy / Earthy / Woodsy / Herbal

Effects	Strength
Peaceful	○ ○ ○ ○ ○
Sleepy	○ ○ ○ ○ ○
Pain Relief	○ ○ ○ ○ ○
Hungry	○ ○ ○ ○ ○
Uplifted	○ ○ ○ ○ ○
Creative	○ ○ ○ ○ ○

Ratings ☆ ☆ ☆ ☆ ☆

Strain

Grower _____ Date _____

Acquired _____ $ _____

| Indica | Hybrid | Sativa |

☐ Flower ☐ Edible ☐ Concentrate

Symptoms Relieved
_____
_____
_____
_____
_____

Sweet · Floral · Spicy · Herbal · Woodsy · Earthy · Sour · Fruity

Notes
_____
_____
_____
_____
_____
_____
_____

Effects	Strength				
Peaceful	○	○	○	○	○
Sleepy	○	○	○	○	○
Pain Relief	○	○	○	○	○
Hungry	○	○	○	○	○
Uplifted	○	○	○	○	○
Creative	○	○	○	○	○

Ratings ☆ ☆ ☆ ☆ ☆

Strain

Grower _____ Date _____

Acquired _____ $ _____

Indica   Hybrid   Sativa

☐ Flower   ☐ Edible   ☐ Concentrate

Sweet · Floral · Spicy · Herbal · Woodsy · Earthy · Sour · Fruity

Symptoms Relieved

_____
_____
_____
_____
_____

Notes

_____
_____
_____
_____
_____
_____

Effects	Strength				
Peaceful	○	○	○	○	○
Sleepy	○	○	○	○	○
Pain Relief	○	○	○	○	○
Hungry	○	○	○	○	○
Uplifted	○	○	○	○	○
Creative	○	○	○	○	○

Ratings ☆ ☆ ☆ ☆ ☆

Strain

Grower _____   Date _____

Acquired _____ $ _____

| Indica | Hybrid | Sativa |

☐ Flower   ☐ Edible   ☐ Concentrate

Symptoms Relieved
_____
_____
_____
_____
_____

Sweet · Fruity · Floral · Sour · Spicy · Earthy · Woodsy · Herbal

Notes
_____
_____
_____
_____
_____
_____
_____

Effects	Strength
Peaceful	○ ○ ○ ○ ○
Sleepy	○ ○ ○ ○ ○
Pain Relief	○ ○ ○ ○ ○
Hungry	○ ○ ○ ○ ○
Uplifted	○ ○ ○ ○ ○
Creative	○ ○ ○ ○ ○

Ratings ☆ ☆ ☆ ☆ ☆

Strain

Grower _____ Date _____

Acquired _____ $ _____

| Indica | Hybrid | Sativa |

☐ Flower ☐ Edible ☐ Concentrate

Sweet · Fruity · Floral · Sour · Spicy · Earthy · Herbal · Woodsy

Symptoms Relieved

_____
_____
_____
_____
_____

Notes

_____
_____
_____
_____
_____
_____

Effects — Strength

- Peaceful ○ ○ ○ ○ ○
- Sleepy ○ ○ ○ ○ ○
- Pain Relief ○ ○ ○ ○ ○
- Hungry ○ ○ ○ ○ ○
- Uplifted ○ ○ ○ ○ ○
- Creative ○ ○ ○ ○ ○

Ratings ☆ ☆ ☆ ☆ ☆

Strain

Grower _____ Date _____

Acquired _____ $ _____

| Indica | Hybrid | Sativa |

☐ Flower ☐ Edible ☐ Concentrate

Symptoms Relieved
_____
_____
_____
_____
_____

Sweet / Floral / Spicy / Herbal / Woodsy / Earthy / Sour / Fruity

Notes
_____
_____
_____
_____
_____
_____

Effects	Strength
Peaceful	○ ○ ○ ○ ○
Sleepy	○ ○ ○ ○ ○
Pain Relief	○ ○ ○ ○ ○
Hungry	○ ○ ○ ○ ○
Uplifted	○ ○ ○ ○ ○
Creative	○ ○ ○ ○ ○

Ratings ☆ ☆ ☆ ☆ ☆

Strain

Grower _____ Date _____

Acquired _____ $ _____

Indica   Hybrid   Sativa

☐ Flower   ☐ Edible   ☐ Concentrate

Symptoms Relieved

_____
_____
_____
_____

Sweet · Floral · Spicy · Herbal · Woodsy · Earthy · Sour · Fruity

Notes

_____
_____
_____
_____
_____
_____
_____

Effects	Strength				
Peaceful	○	○	○	○	○
Sleepy	○	○	○	○	○
Pain Relief	○	○	○	○	○
Hungry	○	○	○	○	○
Uplifted	○	○	○	○	○
Creative	○	○	○	○	○

Ratings ☆ ☆ ☆ ☆ ☆

Strain

Grower _____ Date _____

Acquired _____ $ _____

| Indica | Hybrid | Sativa |

☐ Flower ☐ Edible ☐ Concentrate

Symptoms Relieved

_____
_____
_____
_____
_____

Sweet
Fruity — Floral
Sour — Spicy
Earthy — Herbal
Woodsy

Notes

_____
_____
_____
_____
_____
_____

Effects	Strength				
Peaceful	○	○	○	○	○
Sleepy	○	○	○	○	○
Pain Relief	○	○	○	○	○
Hungry	○	○	○	○	○
Uplifted	○	○	○	○	○
Creative	○	○	○	○	○

Ratings ☆ ☆ ☆ ☆ ☆

Strain

Grower _____ Date _____

Acquired _____ $ _____

| Indica | Hybrid | Sativa |

☐ Flower   ☐ Edible   ☐ Concentrate

Symptoms Relieved

_____
_____
_____
_____

Sweet · Fruity · Floral · Sour · Spicy · Earthy · Herbal · Woodsy

Notes

_____
_____
_____
_____
_____

Effects	Strength				
Peaceful	○	○	○	○	○
Sleepy	○	○	○	○	○
Pain Relief	○	○	○	○	○
Hungry	○	○	○	○	○
Uplifted	○	○	○	○	○
Creative	○	○	○	○	○

Ratings ☆ ☆ ☆ ☆ ☆

Strain

Grower _____   Date _____

Acquired _____ $ _____

| Indica | Hybrid | Sativa |

☐ Flower ☐ Edible ☐ Concentrate

Symptoms Relieved
_____
_____
_____
_____
_____

Sweet · Floral · Spicy · Herbal · Woodsy · Earthy · Sour · Fruity

Notes
_____
_____
_____
_____
_____
_____
_____

Effects	Strength				
Peaceful	○	○	○	○	○
Sleepy	○	○	○	○	○
Pain Relief	○	○	○	○	○
Hungry	○	○	○	○	○
Uplifted	○	○	○	○	○
Creative	○	○	○	○	○

Ratings ☆ ☆ ☆ ☆ ☆

Strain

Grower _____ Date _____

Acquired _____ $ _____

| Indica | Hybrid | Sativa |

☐ Flower   ☐ Edible   ☐ Concentrate

Symptoms Relieved

_____
_____
_____
_____

Sweet
Fruity   Floral
Sour   Spicy
Earthy   Herbal
Woodsy

Notes

_____
_____
_____
_____
_____

Effects	Strength
Peaceful	○ ○ ○ ○ ○
Sleepy	○ ○ ○ ○ ○
Pain Relief	○ ○ ○ ○ ○
Hungry	○ ○ ○ ○ ○
Uplifted	○ ○ ○ ○ ○
Creative	○ ○ ○ ○ ○

Ratings ☆ ☆ ☆ ☆ ☆

Strain

Grower _____   Date _____

Acquired _____ $ _____

| Indica | Hybrid | Sativa |

☐ Flower   ☐ Edible   ☐ Concentrate

Symptoms Relieved

_____
_____
_____
_____
_____

Sweet · Fruity · Floral · Sour · Spicy · Earthy · Woodsy · Herbal

Notes

_____
_____
_____
_____
_____
_____

Effects	Strength				
Peaceful	○	○	○	○	○
Sleepy	○	○	○	○	○
Pain Relief	○	○	○	○	○
Hungry	○	○	○	○	○
Uplifted	○	○	○	○	○
Creative	○	○	○	○	○

Ratings ☆ ☆ ☆ ☆ ☆

Strain

Grower _____ Date _____

Acquired _____ $ _____

| Indica | Hybrid | Sativa |

☐ Flower ☐ Edible ☐ Concentrate

Sweet
Fruity   Floral
Sour   Spicy
Earthy   Herbal
Woodsy

Symptoms Relieved

_____
_____
_____
_____

Notes

_____
_____
_____
_____
_____

Effects	Strength
Peaceful	○ ○ ○ ○ ○
Sleepy	○ ○ ○ ○ ○
Pain Relief	○ ○ ○ ○ ○
Hungry	○ ○ ○ ○ ○
Uplifted	○ ○ ○ ○ ○
Creative	○ ○ ○ ○ ○

Ratings ☆ ☆ ☆ ☆ ☆

Strain

Grower _____ Date _____

Acquired _____ $ _____

| Indica | Hybrid | Sativa |

☐ Flower   ☐ Edible   ☐ Concentrate

Symptoms Relieved

_____
_____
_____
_____
_____

Sweet · Floral · Spicy · Herbal · Woodsy · Earthy · Sour · Fruity

Notes

_____
_____
_____
_____
_____
_____

Effects	Strength				
Peaceful	○	○	○	○	○
Sleepy	○	○	○	○	○
Pain Relief	○	○	○	○	○
Hungry	○	○	○	○	○
Uplifted	○	○	○	○	○
Creative	○	○	○	○	○

Ratings ☆ ☆ ☆ ☆ ☆

Strain

Grower _____ Date _____

Acquired _____ $ _____

| Indica | Hybrid | Sativa |

☐ Flower   ☐ Edible   ☐ Concentrate

Symptoms Relieved

_____
_____
_____
_____

Sweet · Floral · Spicy · Herbal · Woodsy · Earthy · Sour · Fruity

Notes

_____
_____
_____
_____
_____

Effects	Strength				
Peaceful	○	○	○	○	○
Sleepy	○	○	○	○	○
Pain Relief	○	○	○	○	○
Hungry	○	○	○	○	○
Uplifted	○	○	○	○	○
Creative	○	○	○	○	○

Ratings ☆ ☆ ☆ ☆ ☆

Strain

Grower _____ Date _____

Acquired _____ $ _____

| Indica | Hybrid | Sativa |

☐ Flower ☐ Edible ☐ Concentrate

Symptoms Relieved

_____
_____
_____
_____
_____

Sweet / Floral / Spicy / Herbal / Woodsy / Earthy / Sour / Fruity

Notes

_____
_____
_____
_____
_____
_____
_____

Effects	Strength				
Peaceful	○	○	○	○	○
Sleepy	○	○	○	○	○
Pain Relief	○	○	○	○	○
Hungry	○	○	○	○	○
Uplifted	○	○	○	○	○
Creative	○	○	○	○	○

Ratings ☆ ☆ ☆ ☆ ☆

Strain

Grower _____ Date _____

Acquired _____ $ _____

| Indica | Hybrid | Sativa |

☐ Flower ☐ Edible ☐ Concentrate

Symptoms Relieved

_____
_____
_____
_____

Notes

_____
_____
_____
_____
_____
_____

Sweet · Fruity · Floral · Sour · Spicy · Earthy · Woodsy · Herbal

Effects	Strength
Peaceful	○ ○ ○ ○ ○
Sleepy	○ ○ ○ ○ ○
Pain Relief	○ ○ ○ ○ ○
Hungry	○ ○ ○ ○ ○
Uplifted	○ ○ ○ ○ ○
Creative	○ ○ ○ ○ ○

Ratings ☆ ☆ ☆ ☆ ☆

Strain

Grower _____ Date _____

Acquired _____ $ _____

| Indica | Hybrid | Sativa |

☐ Flower ☐ Edible ☐ Concentrate

Sweet · Floral · Spicy · Herbal · Woodsy · Earthy · Sour · Fruity

Symptoms Relieved

_____
_____
_____
_____
_____

Notes

_____
_____
_____
_____
_____
_____

Effects	Strength				
Peaceful	○	○	○	○	○
Sleepy	○	○	○	○	○
Pain Relief	○	○	○	○	○
Hungry	○	○	○	○	○
Uplifted	○	○	○	○	○
Creative	○	○	○	○	○

Ratings ☆ ☆ ☆ ☆ ☆

Strain

Grower _____   Date _____

Acquired _____ $ _____

Indica   Hybrid   Sativa

☐ Flower ☐ Edible ☐ Concentrate

Symptoms Relieved

_____
_____
_____
_____

Sweet / Fruity / Floral / Sour / Spicy / Earthy / Woodsy / Herbal

Notes

_____
_____
_____
_____
_____
_____

Effects	Strength				
Peaceful	○	○	○	○	○
Sleepy	○	○	○	○	○
Pain Relief	○	○	○	○	○
Hungry	○	○	○	○	○
Uplifted	○	○	○	○	○
Creative	○	○	○	○	○

Ratings ☆ ☆ ☆ ☆ ☆

Strain

Grower _____ Date _____

Acquired _____ $ _____

Indica   Hybrid   Sativa

☐ Flower   ☐ Edible   ☐ Concentrate

Symptoms Relieved

_____
_____
_____
_____
_____

Sweet · Fruity · Floral · Sour · Spicy · Earthy · Herbal · Woodsy

Notes

_____
_____
_____
_____
_____

Effects	Strength				
Peaceful	○	○	○	○	○
Sleepy	○	○	○	○	○
Pain Relief	○	○	○	○	○
Hungry	○	○	○	○	○
Uplifted	○	○	○	○	○
Creative	○	○	○	○	○

Ratings ☆ ☆ ☆ ☆ ☆

Strain

Grower _____   Date _____

Acquired _____ $ _____

| Indica | Hybrid | Sativa |

☐ Flower   ☐ Edible   ☐ Concentrate

Symptoms Relieved

_____
_____
_____
_____
_____

Sweet · Fruity · Floral · Sour · Spicy · Earthy · Woodsy · Herbal

Notes

_____
_____
_____
_____
_____
_____
_____

Effects	Strength				
Peaceful	○	○	○	○	○
Sleepy	○	○	○	○	○
Pain Relief	○	○	○	○	○
Hungry	○	○	○	○	○
Uplifted	○	○	○	○	○
Creative	○	○	○	○	○

Ratings ☆ ☆ ☆ ☆ ☆

Strain

Grower _____ Date _____

Acquired _____ $ _____

| Indica | Hybrid | Sativa |

☐ Flower ☐ Edible ☐ Concentrate

Symptoms Relieved
_____
_____
_____
_____
_____

Sweet
Fruity / Floral
Sour / Spicy
Earthy / Herbal
Woodsy

Notes
_____
_____
_____
_____
_____
_____

Effects	Strength				
Peaceful	○	○	○	○	○
Sleepy	○	○	○	○	○
Pain Relief	○	○	○	○	○
Hungry	○	○	○	○	○
Uplifted	○	○	○	○	○
Creative	○	○	○	○	○

Ratings ☆ ☆ ☆ ☆ ☆

Strain

Grower _____   Date _____

Acquired _____ $ _____

| Indica | Hybrid | Sativa |

☐ Flower   ☐ Edible   ☐ Concentrate

Symptoms Relieved

_____
_____
_____
_____
_____

Sweet / Fruity / Floral / Sour / Spicy / Earthy / Woodsy / Herbal

Notes

_____
_____
_____
_____
_____

Effects	Strength				
Peaceful	○	○	○	○	○
Sleepy	○	○	○	○	○
Pain Relief	○	○	○	○	○
Hungry	○	○	○	○	○
Uplifted	○	○	○	○	○
Creative	○	○	○	○	○

Ratings ☆ ☆ ☆ ☆ ☆

Strain

Grower _____ Date _____

Acquired _____ $ _____

| Indica | Hybrid | Sativa |

☐ Flower   ☐ Edible   ☐ Concentrate

Symptoms Relieved
_____
_____
_____
_____
_____

Sweet / Fruity / Floral / Sour / Spicy / Earthy / Woodsy / Herbal

Notes
_____
_____
_____
_____
_____
_____

Effects	Strength				
Peaceful	○	○	○	○	○
Sleepy	○	○	○	○	○
Pain Relief	○	○	○	○	○
Hungry	○	○	○	○	○
Uplifted	○	○	○	○	○
Creative	○	○	○	○	○

Ratings ☆ ☆ ☆ ☆ ☆

Strain

Grower _____ Date _____

Acquired _____ $ _____

| Indica | Hybrid | Sativa |

☐ Flower   ☐ Edible   ☐ Concentrate

Symptoms Relieved

_____
_____
_____
_____
_____

Sweet · Fruity · Floral · Sour · Spicy · Earthy · Woodsy · Herbal

Notes

_____
_____
_____
_____
_____
_____

Effects	Strength
Peaceful	○ ○ ○ ○ ○
Sleepy	○ ○ ○ ○ ○
Pain Relief	○ ○ ○ ○ ○
Hungry	○ ○ ○ ○ ○
Uplifted	○ ○ ○ ○ ○
Creative	○ ○ ○ ○ ○

Ratings ☆ ☆ ☆ ☆ ☆

Strain

Grower _____ Date _____

Acquired _____ $ _____

Indica   Hybrid   Sativa

☐ Flower   ☐ Edible   ☐ Concentrate

Symptoms Relieved
_____
_____
_____
_____
_____

Sweet / Fruity / Floral / Sour / Spicy / Earthy / Herbal / Woodsy

Notes
_____
_____
_____
_____
_____

Effects	Strength				
Peaceful	○	○	○	○	○
Sleepy	○	○	○	○	○
Pain Relief	○	○	○	○	○
Hungry	○	○	○	○	○
Uplifted	○	○	○	○	○
Creative	○	○	○	○	○

Ratings ☆ ☆ ☆ ☆ ☆

Strain

Grower _____ Date _____

Acquired _____ $ _____

| Indica | Hybrid | Sativa |

☐ Flower ☐ Edible ☐ Concentrate

Symptoms Relieved
_____
_____
_____
_____

Sweet / Fruity / Floral / Sour / Spicy / Earthy / Herbal / Woodsy

Notes
_____
_____
_____
_____
_____

Effects	Strength				
Peaceful	○	○	○	○	○
Sleepy	○	○	○	○	○
Pain Relief	○	○	○	○	○
Hungry	○	○	○	○	○
Uplifted	○	○	○	○	○
Creative	○	○	○	○	○

Ratings ☆ ☆ ☆ ☆ ☆

Strain

Grower _____ Date _____

Acquired _____ $ _____

| Indica | Hybrid | Sativa |

☐ Flower ☐ Edible ☐ Concentrate

Flavor wheel: Sweet, Floral, Spicy, Herbal, Woodsy, Earthy, Sour, Fruity

Symptoms Relieved

_____
_____
_____
_____
_____

Notes

_____
_____
_____
_____
_____
_____

Effects	Strength
Peaceful	○ ○ ○ ○ ○
Sleepy	○ ○ ○ ○ ○
Pain Relief	○ ○ ○ ○ ○
Hungry	○ ○ ○ ○ ○
Uplifted	○ ○ ○ ○ ○
Creative	○ ○ ○ ○ ○

Ratings ☆ ☆ ☆ ☆ ☆

Strain

Grower _____ Date _____

Acquired _____ $ _____

| Indica | Hybrid | Sativa |

☐ Flower   ☐ Edible   ☐ Concentrate

Symptoms Relieved

_____
_____
_____
_____

Notes

_____
_____
_____
_____
_____
_____

Sweet · Floral · Spicy · Herbal · Woodsy · Earthy · Sour · Fruity

Effects	Strength
Peaceful	○ ○ ○ ○ ○
Sleepy	○ ○ ○ ○ ○
Pain Relief	○ ○ ○ ○ ○
Hungry	○ ○ ○ ○ ○
Uplifted	○ ○ ○ ○ ○
Creative	○ ○ ○ ○ ○

Ratings ☆ ☆ ☆ ☆ ☆

Strain

Grower _____ Date _____

Acquired _____ $ _____

| Indica | Hybrid | Sativa |

☐ Flower ☐ Edible ☐ Concentrate

Symptoms Relieved

_____
_____
_____
_____
_____

Sweet / Fruity / Floral / Sour / Spicy / Earthy / Woodsy / Herbal

Notes

_____
_____
_____
_____
_____
_____

Effects	Strength				
Peaceful	○	○	○	○	○
Sleepy	○	○	○	○	○
Pain Relief	○	○	○	○	○
Hungry	○	○	○	○	○
Uplifted	○	○	○	○	○
Creative	○	○	○	○	○

Ratings ☆ ☆ ☆ ☆ ☆

Strain

Grower _____ Date _____

Acquired _____ $ _____

| Indica | Hybrid | Sativa |

☐ Flower ☐ Edible ☐ Concentrate

Symptoms Relieved

_____
_____
_____
_____

Sweet / Fruity / Floral / Sour / Spicy / Earthy / Woodsy / Herbal

Notes

_____
_____
_____
_____
_____
_____

Effects	Strength
Peaceful	○ ○ ○ ○ ○
Sleepy	○ ○ ○ ○ ○
Pain Relief	○ ○ ○ ○ ○
Hungry	○ ○ ○ ○ ○
Uplifted	○ ○ ○ ○ ○
Creative	○ ○ ○ ○ ○

Ratings ☆ ☆ ☆ ☆ ☆

Strain

Grower _____ Date _____

Acquired _____ $ _____

Indica   Hybrid   Sativa

☐ Flower   ☐ Edible   ☐ Concentrate

Symptoms Relieved

_____
_____
_____
_____
_____

Sweet
Fruity   Floral
Sour   Spicy
Earthy   Herbal
Woodsy

Notes

_____
_____
_____
_____
_____
_____

Effects	Strength				
Peaceful	○	○	○	○	○
Sleepy	○	○	○	○	○
Pain Relief	○	○	○	○	○
Hungry	○	○	○	○	○
Uplifted	○	○	○	○	○
Creative	○	○	○	○	○

Ratings ☆ ☆ ☆ ☆ ☆

Strain

Grower _____ Date _____

Acquired _____ $ _____

| Indica | Hybrid | Sativa |

☐ Flower ☐ Edible ☐ Concentrate

Sweet
Fruity   Floral
Sour   Spicy
Earthy   Herbal
Woodsy

Symptoms Relieved

_____
_____
_____
_____
_____

Notes

_____
_____
_____
_____
_____
_____

Effects	Strength				
Peaceful	○	○	○	○	○
Sleepy	○	○	○	○	○
Pain Relief	○	○	○	○	○
Hungry	○	○	○	○	○
Uplifted	○	○	○	○	○
Creative	○	○	○	○	○

Ratings ☆ ☆ ☆ ☆ ☆

Strain

Grower _____ Date _____

Acquired _____ $ _____

| Indica | Hybrid | Sativa |

☐ Flower   ☐ Edible   ☐ Concentrate

Symptoms Relieved

_____
_____
_____
_____
_____

Sweet
Fruity   Floral
Sour   Spicy
Earthy   Herbal
Woodsy

Notes

_____
_____
_____
_____
_____
_____

Effects	Strength
Peaceful	○ ○ ○ ○ ○
Sleepy	○ ○ ○ ○ ○
Pain Relief	○ ○ ○ ○ ○
Hungry	○ ○ ○ ○ ○
Uplifted	○ ○ ○ ○ ○
Creative	○ ○ ○ ○ ○

Ratings ☆ ☆ ☆ ☆ ☆

Strain

Grower _____   Date _____

Acquired _____ $ _____

| Indica | Hybrid | Sativa |

☐ Flower ☐ Edible ☐ Concentrate

Symptoms Relieved

_____
_____
_____
_____

Sweet · Floral · Spicy · Herbal · Woodsy · Earthy · Sour · Fruity

Notes

_____
_____
_____
_____
_____

Effects	Strength				
Peaceful	○	○	○	○	○
Sleepy	○	○	○	○	○
Pain Relief	○	○	○	○	○
Hungry	○	○	○	○	○
Uplifted	○	○	○	○	○
Creative	○	○	○	○	○

Ratings ☆ ☆ ☆ ☆ ☆

Strain

Grower _____ Date _____

Acquired _____ $ _____

| Indica | Hybrid | Sativa |

☐ Flower   ☐ Edible   ☐ Concentrate

Symptoms Relieved

_____
_____
_____
_____

Sweet · Fruity · Floral · Sour · Spicy · Earthy · Herbal · Woodsy

Notes

_____
_____
_____
_____
_____

Effects	Strength
Peaceful	○ ○ ○ ○ ○
Sleepy	○ ○ ○ ○ ○
Pain Relief	○ ○ ○ ○ ○
Hungry	○ ○ ○ ○ ○
Uplifted	○ ○ ○ ○ ○
Creative	○ ○ ○ ○ ○

Ratings ☆ ☆ ☆ ☆ ☆

Strain

Grower _____ Date _____

Acquired _____ $ _____

Indica   Hybrid   Sativa

☐ Flower   ☐ Edible   ☐ Concentrate

Symptoms Relieved

_____
_____
_____
_____
_____

Sweet / Floral / Spicy / Herbal / Woodsy / Earthy / Sour / Fruity

Notes

_____
_____
_____
_____
_____
_____
_____

Effects	Strength				
Peaceful	○	○	○	○	○
Sleepy	○	○	○	○	○
Pain Relief	○	○	○	○	○
Hungry	○	○	○	○	○
Uplifted	○	○	○	○	○
Creative	○	○	○	○	○

Ratings ☆ ☆ ☆ ☆ ☆

Strain

Grower _____ Date _____

Acquired _____ $ _____

| Indica | Hybrid | Sativa |

☐ Flower ☐ Edible ☐ Concentrate

Symptoms Relieved

_____
_____
_____
_____

Sweet
Fruity   Floral
Sour   Spicy
Earthy   Herbal
Woodsy

Notes

_____
_____
_____
_____
_____

Effects	Strength				
Peaceful	○	○	○	○	○
Sleepy	○	○	○	○	○
Pain Relief	○	○	○	○	○
Hungry	○	○	○	○	○
Uplifted	○	○	○	○	○
Creative	○	○	○	○	○

Ratings ☆ ☆ ☆ ☆ ☆

Strain

Grower _____ Date _____

Acquired _____ $ _____

| Indica | Hybrid | Sativa |

☐ Flower ☐ Edible ☐ Concentrate

Symptoms Relieved

_____
_____
_____
_____
_____

Sweet
Fruity   Floral
Sour   Spicy
Earthy   Herbal
Woodsy

Notes

_____
_____
_____
_____
_____
_____
_____

Effects	Strength
Peaceful	○ ○ ○ ○ ○
Sleepy	○ ○ ○ ○ ○
Pain Relief	○ ○ ○ ○ ○
Hungry	○ ○ ○ ○ ○
Uplifted	○ ○ ○ ○ ○
Creative	○ ○ ○ ○ ○

Ratings ☆ ☆ ☆ ☆ ☆

Strain

Grower _____   Date _____

Acquired _____ $ _____

| Indica | Hybrid | Sativa |

☐ Flower   ☐ Edible   ☐ Concentrate

Symptoms Relieved

_____
_____
_____
_____

Flavor wheel: Sweet, Floral, Spicy, Herbal, Woodsy, Earthy, Sour, Fruity

Notes

_____
_____
_____
_____
_____

Effects	Strength				
Peaceful	○	○	○	○	○
Sleepy	○	○	○	○	○
Pain Relief	○	○	○	○	○
Hungry	○	○	○	○	○
Uplifted	○	○	○	○	○
Creative	○	○	○	○	○

Ratings ☆ ☆ ☆ ☆ ☆

Strain

Grower _____   Date _____

Acquired _____ $ _____

| Indica | Hybrid | Sativa |

☐ Flower   ☐ Edible   ☐ Concentrate

Symptoms Relieved

_____
_____
_____
_____
_____

Sweet · Fruity · Floral · Sour · Spicy · Earthy · Herbal · Woodsy

Notes

_____
_____
_____
_____
_____
_____

Effects	Strength				
Peaceful	○	○	○	○	○
Sleepy	○	○	○	○	○
Pain Relief	○	○	○	○	○
Hungry	○	○	○	○	○
Uplifted	○	○	○	○	○
Creative	○	○	○	○	○

Ratings ☆ ☆ ☆ ☆ ☆

Strain

Grower _____ Date _____

Acquired _____ $ _____

| Indica | Hybrid | Sativa |

☐ Flower   ☐ Edible   ☐ Concentrate

Symptoms Relieved

_____
_____
_____
_____

Flavor wheel: Sweet, Floral, Spicy, Herbal, Woodsy, Earthy, Sour, Fruity

Notes

_____
_____
_____
_____
_____
_____

Effects	Strength				
Peaceful	○	○	○	○	○
Sleepy	○	○	○	○	○
Pain Relief	○	○	○	○	○
Hungry	○	○	○	○	○
Uplifted	○	○	○	○	○
Creative	○	○	○	○	○

Ratings ☆ ☆ ☆ ☆ ☆

Strain

Grower _____   Date _____

Acquired _____ $ _____

| Indica | Hybrid | Sativa |

☐ Flower   ☐ Edible   ☐ Concentrate

Sweet
Fruity   Floral
Sour   Spicy
Earthy   Herbal
Woodsy

Symptoms Relieved

_____
_____
_____
_____

Notes

_____
_____
_____
_____
_____
_____

Effects	Strength
Peaceful	○ ○ ○ ○ ○
Sleepy	○ ○ ○ ○ ○
Pain Relief	○ ○ ○ ○ ○
Hungry	○ ○ ○ ○ ○
Uplifted	○ ○ ○ ○ ○
Creative	○ ○ ○ ○ ○

Ratings ☆ ☆ ☆ ☆ ☆